DEFEATING PARKINSON'S DISEASE WITH EXPERT GUIDANCE

Ultimate Solution Handbook For Patients, Guardians Or Family To Understand, Manage, Treat, Prevent, Reverse Symptoms And Live Well

DR. POTTER WHITLEY

Copyright © 2023 by Dr. Potter Whitley

DISCLAIMER:

This book's contents are meant to be used solely for informative purposes. The information should not be used as a replacement for expert medical advice, diagnosis, or care.

The information contained in this book is accurate and reliable, having been verified by the author to the best of his ability. Nevertheless, the author disclaims all express and implied representations and warranties regarding the availability, correctness, appropriateness, completeness, and reliability of the material provided here. You bear full responsibility for any reliance you may have on such material.

For informational purposes, this book may make reference to or mention of certain people, things, websites, organizations, or other names. The author has no connection to, endorsement from, or recommendation for these organizations. The author's approval or validation is not implied by the inclusion of these references.

Any direct, indirect, incidental, special, or consequential damages resulting from using or not being able to use the material in this book are not covered by the author's liability policy. For medical advice and counsel particular to their circumstances, readers are advised to check with experienced healthcare specialists.

The content, materials, and information in this book are subject to change at any time without prior notice, at the author's discretion. The text may contain errors or omissions for which the author is not responsible.

By reading this book, you understand and accept the conditions of this disclaimer.

THE REASON BEHIND THIS BOOK

In the field of Parkinson's disease literature, "Defeating Parkinson's Disease With Expert Guidance" is a priceless resource. This book begins with an extensive introduction that sets the stage for comprehending the nuances of this neurological illness. Using a thorough investigation, the work highlights the critical function that professional advice serves in negotiating the difficulties presented by Parkinson's disease, underscoring the need for patients and their carers to seek professional help.

The review of Parkinson's disease explores the disease's past and peels back the layers to reveal its causes, risk factors, symptoms, and course. This book helps readers understand the complexities of this complicated illness by offering a nuanced understanding. The text examines the roles of neurologists in the management of Parkinson's disease, recognizing the significance of medical professionals and highlighting the advantages of a collaborative healthcare approach as well as the importance of early diagnosis.

Treatment options available today are examined in detail, including drugs, surgery, and physical therapy. This book broadens its scope to include lifestyle factors in the management of Parkinson's disease, emphasizing the benefits of stress reduction, good diet, and exercise. Slickly navigating cutting-edge techniques such as gene therapy, stem cell research, and deep brain stimulation, it offers an overview of the landscape of developing therapeutics.

A major focus is psychosocial support for patients and caregivers, which addresses issues related to mental health, the value of support networks, and striking a careful balance between autonomy and help. This book offers helpful advice on coping mechanisms for day-to-day living, including home adaptations, adaptive technology, and maintaining quality of life.

Mind-body techniques, integrative medicine, and complementary and alternative therapies are all included in the holistic approaches to Parkinson's care. This book explores ongoing research, clinical trials, and promising breakthroughs as the story progresses, giving patients hope and promoting patient advocacy in the constantly changing field of Parkinson's research.

In this book, the empowerment of the Parkinson's community is turned into a call to action, with a focus on advocacy, education, and public awareness raising. The significance of developing a network of support and fostering a sense of cohesion and strength among the Parkinson's community is emphasized in the conclusion. Essentially, this book is more than just a manual; it is a source of information and encouragement, giving its readers the skills and understanding required to face and overcome the obstacles presented by Parkinson's disease.

TABLE OF CONTENT

CHAPTER ONE

INTRODUCTION
Comprehending Parkinson's Disease

Research and medical exploration into Parkinson's disease, a progressive neurodegenerative disorder, have been extensive. Investigating the underlying biological mechanisms of this condition is essential to understanding its complexities. Fundamentally, Parkinson's disease is defined by the slow deterioration of neurons in the brain's substantia nigra region that produce dopamine. As a result of this neural breakdown, dopamine, a neurotransmitter essential for fluid, and coordinated muscle movements, is deficient. The classic Parkinson's disease motor symptoms, including bradykinesia, rigidity, tremors, and postural instability, are manifestations of this deficiency.

Parkinson's disease is known to impact several non-motor functions in addition to its motor symptoms, such as cognitive decline, autonomic dysfunction, and psychological disorders. Because of the disease's complexity, creating a successful treatment plan requires a thorough understanding of its pathology. To identify potential therapeutic targets, scientists are examining the role that age, environment, and genetic factors play in the development and progression of Parkinson's disease.

Furthermore, Parkinson's affects not just the person with the diagnosis but also the lives of family members and caregivers. The difficulties presented by the illness highlight how urgent it is to comprehend its biological causes and create comprehensive strategies to improve the lives of those who are impacted.

Importance of Professional Advice

The importance of professional advice in the complicated world of managing Parkinson's disease cannot be emphasized. The complex web of symptoms, therapies, and lifestyle modifications must be navigated with the knowledge and skills of medical professionals skilled in neurology, rehabilitation, and related disciplines. These professionals are essential in making precise diagnoses, creating individualized treatment programs, and providing patients and their families with continuous support.

When it comes to customizing interventions to meet the specific needs of every person, expert advice is especially important. Every patient experiences Parkinson's disease differently, necessitating a personalized and complex approach to treatment. Recognizing that a one-size-fits-all approach is insufficient, neurologists, physical therapists, occupational therapists, and other specialists work together to address the various challenges presented by the disease.

Additionally, professional guidance guarantees that patients have access to the newest and most efficient interventions as research progresses and new treatment modalities emerge. This entails keeping up with medical advancements as well as assessing how applicable they are to particular situations.

Parkinson's disease specialists are at the forefront of converting scientific discoveries into observable benefits for patients.

Expert advice goes beyond the clinical setting to include educating patients' support systems about Parkinson's disease. People are better able to take an active role in their care journey when they are aware of the condition, how it progresses, and the available management options. Under the direction of a specialist, the psychological and emotional aspects of having Parkinson's disease are also addressed, promoting coping mechanisms and resilience.

In summary, the foundation of successful management is a thorough understanding of Parkinson's disease combined with the advice of seasoned professionals. The convergence of knowledge and experience creates opportunities for improved quality of life and a more all-encompassing strategy for addressing the complex issues raised by Parkinson's disease.

CHAPTER TWO

AN OVERVIEW OF PARKINSON'S DISEASE
Historical Angle:

The history of Parkinson's disease is extensive and dates back thousands of years. The oldest documented accounts of Parkinson-like symptoms come from prehistoric societies. However, the illness was not recognized as a separate medical entity until the early 19th century. In his groundbreaking work "An Essay on the Shaking Palsy," published in 1817, British physician James Parkinson described the disease's hallmark tremors, stiffness, and poor balance. The understanding and categorization of Parkinson's disease were established by this ground-breaking document.

In the decades that followed, developments in both medicine and technology deepened our understanding of the neurodegenerative character of the illness. A turning point in the development of Parkinson's disease research and therapy was the discovery that dopamine deficiency, specifically in the basal ganglia, is a major contributor to the pathophysiology of Parkinson's disease. The discovery of levodopa, a dopamine precursor, in the 1960s transformed treatment modalities and markedly enhanced the quality of life for Parkinson's patients.

A closer look at the historical account reveals that the complexity of Parkinson's disease has been gradually revealed throughout the understanding process. The historical view of Parkinson's disease illustrates the scientific community's tenacity in the face of a complex and multidimensional illness, from the disease's initial clinical observations by Parkinson to the current molecular-level studies.

Reasons and Danger Factors:

Parkinson's disease is a multifactorial disorder, meaning that environmental and genetic factors interact intricately to influence the disease's onset. Although the precise cause of Parkinson's disease is still unknown, a great deal of research has revealed potential causes and risk factors.

There is a strong genetic component to the illness, with some genetic mutations making a person more susceptible to it. Gene mutations including SNCA, LRRK2, and PARKIN have been linked to familial cases of Parkinson's disease, offering important new information about the genetic components of the illness. It is important to remember, though, that most cases of Parkinson's are sporadic and do not appear to have a clear genetic cause.

The risk profile is also influenced by environmental variables. Parkinson's disease incidence has been related to exposure to specific toxins, including herbicides and pesticides. A history of particular occupations like farming or welding, as well as head injuries, may also increase the risk.

Deciphering the intricate web of factors contributing to Parkinson's disease requires an understanding of how genetic predisposition and environmental triggers interact. The goal of ongoing research is to clarify the complex pathways that result in the death of neurons that produce dopamine, as this will lay the groundwork for focused treatment approaches and prophylactic measures.

Signs and Development:

A variety of motor and non-motor symptoms that appear gradually over time are indicative of Parkinson's disease. Tremors, bradykinesia (slowness of movement), rigidity, and postural instability are the hallmark motor symptoms. The substantia nigra, a crucial area of the brain, is home to dopamine-producing neurons that are degenerating, which causes the symptoms collectively referred to as parkinsonism.

People may develop a variety of non-motor symptoms that have a substantial impact on their quality of life as the disease advances. These may consist of autonomic dysfunction, mood swings, sleep issues, and cognitive impairment. The diagnosis and treatment of Parkinson's disease are frequently complicated by the non-motor symptoms, underscoring the importance of an all-encompassing, multidisciplinary approach.

Parkinson's disease progresses very differently in each person; some may see a more rapid deterioration in function, while others may see a relatively slow decline. A framework for comprehending the progressive nature of Parkinson's disease is provided by the Hoehn and Yahr scale, which is frequently used to evaluate the severity of the disease's symptoms.

Researchers look into the underlying neurobiology to understand the complexities of symptom development and progression. They are looking for biomarkers that could help with early diagnosis and intervention. Technological developments in imaging and molecular biology are expanding our knowledge of the dynamic processes occurring in the brain and opening doors to customized treatment plans catered

to the specific requirements of Parkinson's disease
patients.

CHAPTER THREE

THE FUNCTION OF HEALTH CARE PRACTITIONERS
Experts in neurology and Parkinson's illness

In the comprehensive care and management of Parkinson's disease (PD), neurologists are essential. Neurologists are specialized medical professionals who are uniquely qualified to comprehend and manage the challenges associated with Parkinson's disease, a complex neurodegenerative disorder characterized by both motor and non-motor symptoms. Their proficiency in the complex mechanisms of the nervous system enables them to accurately diagnose, treat, and monitor the advancement of Parkinson's disease.

Accurate diagnosis is one of the neurologists' main duties when it comes to Parkinson's. Due to the subtle nature of its symptoms, Parkinson's disease (PD) is frequently difficult to definitively diagnose in its early stages.

To reach a definitive diagnosis, neurologists utilize a range of methods including clinical assessments, evaluations of the patient's medical history, and occasionally sophisticated imaging techniques. They can differentiate Parkinson's from other conditions that may present with similar symptoms thanks to their specialized knowledge, which guarantees that patients receive the right support and interventions.

Neurologists are the people with Parkinson's disease's principal point of contact after a diagnosis. Together with other medical specialists, they create individualized treatment programs that take into account the disease's non-motor as well as motor components. These plans typically include lifestyle counseling, physical therapy, and medication management. Additionally, neurologists are essential in tracking the course of Parkinson's disease and modifying treatment plans as necessary to maximize patient outcomes.

Neurologists make a substantial contribution to ongoing research and advancements in Parkinson's treatment, in addition to providing clinical care. Their participation in research projects, clinical trials, and interdisciplinary teams advances our knowledge and therapeutic alternatives. Essentially, neurologists are the front-line experts in the fight against Parkinson's disease because they combine clinical expertise with a dedication to furthering scientific understanding for the betterment of their patients.

The Value of Timely Diagnosis

For multiple reasons, early detection of Parkinson's disease is critical and can significantly change the course of a patient's life. Early diagnosis and treatment not only maximize the efficacy of currently available therapies but also facilitate the development and application of strategies aimed at enhancing the general quality of life for Parkinson's patients.

First of all, timely initiation of appropriate medical interventions is made possible by early diagnosis.

Although there isn't a known cure for Parkinson's disease, there are several drugs and treatments that can effectively control symptoms and halt the disease's progression. Early implementation of these treatments can improve mobility, delay the onset of complications, and significantly reduce motor symptoms. Early intervention may also make it possible for patients to take part in experimental treatments and clinical trials, which may give them access to state-of-the-art treatments.

Second, the execution of thorough, multidisciplinary care plans is made easier by early diagnosis. Healthcare providers can work together to treat Parkinson's disease not only for its motor symptoms but also for its non-motor ones, like mental and cognitive problems. This all-encompassing strategy guarantees that the various difficulties brought on by Parkinson's are handled in a coordinated way and enhances the general well-being of the patient.

Furthermore, early diagnosis gives Parkinson's patients and their families the ability to actively manage the illness. Early diagnosis and treatment planning facilitate improved living space adaptation, better planning, and the integration of lifestyle modifications that can improve day-to-day functioning. Early implementation of education and support services can provide patients and caregivers with the necessary tools to manage the social, emotional, and physical aspects of living with Parkinson's disease.

In conclusion, it is impossible to overestimate the significance of an early diagnosis of Parkinson's disease. It maximizes the effectiveness of treatment, lays the groundwork for prompt and focused interventions, and enhances the general quality of life for individuals with this neurodegenerative illness.

The Collaborative Healthcare Method

Due to the intricate nature of Parkinson's disease, a collaborative approach to healthcare is required, in which different medical specialists collaborate to address the unique needs of patients with the disease.

To create a comprehensive and customized care plan, this collaborative model brings together neurologists, primary care physicians, physical therapists, occupational therapists, speech therapists, social workers, and other specialists, each of whom brings a unique set of skills to the table.

As the principal specialists in charge of Parkinson's care, neurologists work in conjunction with other medical specialists to guarantee a comprehensive approach to treatment. They collaborate closely with physical therapists to create exercise plans that improve mobility and target particular motor symptoms. Occupational therapists assist in improving functional independence by addressing difficulties associated with daily activities, offering adaptive strategies, and endorsing assistive devices.

When it comes to treating the speech and swallowing issues that can accompany Parkinson's disease, speech therapists are essential. Their knowledge lowers the possibility of problems associated with eating and drinking while facilitating efficient communication. Social workers play a critical role in addressing the psychosocial effects of Parkinson's on the affected person and their support system, offering emotional support, and putting patients and families in touch with local resources.

The collaborative approach to healthcare goes beyond the boundaries of clinical practice. Scientists and researchers conduct studies, and clinical trials, and create new interventions to add to the body of knowledge. The collaborative model is informed and enhanced by this ongoing research, which guarantees that medical professionals are aware of the most recent developments in Parkinson's treatment.

Caregivers and family members are also essential components of the collaborative healthcare model. Their understanding of the day-to-day struggles that people with Parkinson's disease face is priceless, and they frequently collaborate closely with medical professionals to put strategies into place that improve the patient's overall care and support.

The collaborative healthcare approach, in its most basic form, acknowledges the complex nature of Parkinson's disease and the need for a team effort to address its complexities. Through the utilization of the skills of various medical specialists and the inclusion of patient and support system viewpoints, this method seeks to offer all-encompassing, patient-focused treatment across the full range of Parkinson's disease.

CHAPTER FOUR

PRESENTLY USED TREATMENT APPROACHES
Pharmaceuticals For Parkinson's Illness:

Parkinson's disease (PD) is a neurodegenerative condition marked by the brain's dopamine-producing neurons gradually dying off. Even though there isn't a cure for Parkinson's disease (PD), drugs are essential for controlling its symptoms and enhancing patients' quality of life. The most popular and effective drug for Parkinson's disease (PD), levodopa, makes up for dopamine deficit in the brain by converting to dopamine. On the other hand, dyskinesias and motor fluctuations may result from prolonged use.

Additional drugs include monoamine oxidase-B (MAO-B) inhibitors, which increase the efficiency of dopamine in the brain, and dopamine agonists, which imitate the effects of dopamine. To manage tremors, doctors may also prescribe anticholinergic medications. However, PD medication management is very patient-specific, with doctors taking the patient's age, overall health, and individual symptoms into account.

Although these drugs are good at relieving symptoms, there may be problems with using them over the long term. Patients' responses can fluctuate, necessitating dosage changes or additional medication. Furthermore, it becomes essential to control side effects like nausea, hallucinations, or insomnia to strike a balance between symptom relief and quality of life.

Surgical Solutions:

When medication alone is not enough to control symptoms, surgical interventions may be a viable option for patients with advanced Parkinson's disease. An established surgical technique called Deep Brain Stimulation (DBS) entails implanting electrodes into particular brain regions and connecting them to a pulse generator positioned beneath the skin. Motor symptoms such as bradykinesia, stiffness, and tremors are significantly relieved by the electrical stimulation, which modifies aberrant nerve signals.

While DBS cannot cure a patient, it can minimize side effects by increasing the effectiveness of medication and lowering the need for higher doses. Candidates for DBS are chosen after a thorough assessment of their general health, cognitive abilities, and medication response. Patients participate in programming sessions after surgery to maximize the benefits of optimal stimulation settings.

DBS is effective, but it's vital to remember that, similar to any surgery, there are risks involved, such as the possibility of infection and hardware-related complications. Its effect on non-motor symptoms is also still being studied.

Further surgical alternatives, like gene therapy and focused ultrasound, are still being investigated in research, providing encouraging treatment options for Parkinson's disease in the future.

Therapies for Rehabilitation:

For those with Parkinson's disease, rehabilitation therapies are essential in addition to medication and surgical procedures. Physical therapy addresses the motor symptoms that have a major impact on day-to-day functioning by focusing on enhancing mobility, balance, and flexibility. The goal of occupational therapy is to improve independence by concentrating on daily living skills like writing, cooking, and clothing. PD is frequently linked to swallowing problems and communication difficulties, which speech therapy can help manage.

In Parkinson's patients, exercise—including strength training and aerobic activities—has been shown to improve motor function and general well-being. It enhances mood and cognitive function in addition to physical function. Popular methods of stimulating the physical and cognitive domains while encouraging neuroplasticity and possibly delaying the course of the disease are dance and music therapy.

Rehab treatments are important because they are customized to meet the needs of each patient, taking into account the stage and particular symptoms of Parkinson's disease. Current studies are investigating novel strategies, such as virtual reality and robotics, to augment the efficacy of rehabilitation interventions and ultimately elevate the standard of living for Parkinson's patients.

CHAPTER FIVE

PARKINSON'S DISEASE MANAGEMENT AND LIFESTYLE
Physical Activity And Exercise In The Treatment Of Parkinson's Disease:

Exercise is essential for Parkinson's disease management because it provides a variety of benefits for improving mental and physical health. Frequent exercise has been demonstrated to reduce a number of Parkinson's symptoms, including tremors, stiffness, and problems with balance. Aerobic exercises can improve general mobility and support cardiovascular health. Examples of these exercises include swimming, cycling, and brisk walking. Strength training exercises also help to address the muscle rigidity that Parkinson's patients frequently experience by improving muscle flexibility and stability.

In addition, workouts like yoga and tai chi that concentrate on enhancing balance and coordination might be especially helpful. In addition to improving physical function, these activities offer a forum for social interaction, which helps counteract the possibility of isolation that comes with a long-term illness such as Parkinson's. It's important to incorporate a variety of activities into your regimen and adjust it to suit your needs and tastes.

It is crucial to include physical activity in the daily schedule. Mobility problems can be accommodated with the help of assistive technologies and adaptive tactics. Under the direction of medical professionals and physical therapists, routine evaluations and modifications to the workout program guarantee that the regimen stays safe and effective over time. By prioritizing a continuous and diverse exercise regimen, individuals with Parkinson's can greatly contribute to their personal well-being and quality of life.

Nutrition and Dietary Considerations in Parkinson's Management:

Nutrition has a significant role in the management of Parkinson's disease, influencing both the course of the ailment and the overall well-being of individuals. While there is no unique "Parkinson's diet," adopting a balanced and nutritious eating plan can significantly impact different aspects of health. Antioxidant-rich foods, such as fruits and vegetables, can help counteract oxidative stress, which is implicated in the neurodegenerative process of Parkinson's.

Moreover, keeping a healthy weight is vital, since obesity can intensify symptoms and contribute to other health concerns. Adequate protein consumption, distributed evenly throughout the day, is a priority due to potential interactions with Parkinson's drugs. Collaborating with a qualified dietitian can assist in customizing nutritional guidelines to individual needs, including considerations such as medication scheduling and potential side effects.

Hydration is another crucial part of nutrition, as Parkinson's drugs may raise the risk of dehydration. Ensuring a sufficient hydration intake helps improve overall health and can lessen some medication-related side effects. Additionally, some patients with Parkinson's may encounter swallowing difficulty, needing modifications in food texture and consistency.

Overall, a tailored and well-balanced approach to nutrition is crucial in controlling Parkinson's disease. Regular meetings with healthcare specialists and dietitians can ensure that dietary regimens are optimized to support both physical health and the effectiveness of medical therapies.

Sleep and Stress Management in Parkinson's Management:

Sleep difficulties and heightened stress levels are significant challenges for persons living with Parkinson's disease. Addressing these difficulties is vital not just for enhancing the overall quality of life but also for potentially impacting the course of the condition. Implementing excellent sleep hygiene routines is paramount. Establishing a consistent sleep schedule, improving the sleep environment, and minimizing stimulants in the evening can lead to better sleep quality.

Stress management is also vital, as heightened stress can increase Parkinson's symptoms. Techniques such as mindfulness meditation, deep breathing exercises, and progressive muscle relaxation can be beneficial in fostering relaxation and reducing stress levels. Engaging in activities that bring joy and relaxation, such as hobbies or spending time in nature, can also help general well-being.

Moreover, developing a robust support system is vital for emotional well-being. Parkinson's disease can be emotionally demanding, and having a network of friends, family, and support groups can provide both practical assistance and emotional support. Regular communication with healthcare specialists ensures that stress and sleep difficulties are addressed holistically, incorporating both medication and lifestyle therapies.

In conclusion, a holistic approach to Parkinson's management that includes attention to exercise, nutrition, sleep, and stress management can considerably enhance the quality of life for persons living with this condition.

By incorporating these lifestyle components into a holistic treatment plan, individuals with Parkinson's can empower themselves to better navigate the obstacles associated with the disease and enhance overall well-being.

CHAPTER SIX

INNOVATIVE APPROACHES AND EMERGING THERAPIES
Deep Brain Stimulation (DBS)

Deep Brain Stimulation (DBS) has emerged as a pioneering and novel treatment in the fight against Parkinson's Disease (PD). PD is a neurodegenerative condition defined by the loss of dopamine-producing neurons in the brain, leading to movement deficits. DBS includes the implantation of electrodes into specific parts of the brain, generally the subthalamic nucleus or the globus pallidus internus. These electrodes deliver electrical impulses that control aberrant brain activity, relieving motor symptoms linked with PD.

One of the primary advantages of DBS is its capacity to give targeted and customizable stimulation. Neurologists can fine-tune the settings of the electrical impulses to improve therapeutic outcomes, minimizing negative effects. This tailored strategy optimizes treatment outcomes and improves the patient's quality of life. DBS is particularly effective for those with advanced PD who may not react well to medicines alone.

Furthermore, continuing research strives to refine and expand the applicability of DBS. Researchers are studying fresh brain targets and upgrading electrode implantation techniques to enhance the precision of stimulation. Additionally, developments in device technology are making DBS systems more efficient, smaller, and capable of extended battery life. These improvements contribute to the overall efficacy and sustainability of DBS as a treatment intervention for PD.

Despite its success, problems exist, such as the necessity for long-term monitoring, potential hardware-related complications, and the tuning of stimulation parameters. However, the ongoing progress of DBS techniques and technologies highlights its potential to change Parkinson's treatment, bringing hope to people affected by this devastating disease.

Stem Cell Research

Stem cell research is a promising area in the effort to defeat Parkinson's Disease. The use of stem cells has tremendous potential for rebuilding damaged or destroyed neurons in the brains of PD patients. Stem cells possess the unusual ability to differentiate into diverse cell types, including dopamine-producing neurons necessary for motor function.

Innovative approaches in stem cell treatment involve transplanting stem cells into the brain to repair damaged cells and restore normal neural function. This regenerative technique offers a fresh way to address the fundamental cause of PD by restoring the dwindling pool of dopamine-producing neurons. Moreover, continuing research focuses on optimizing the procurement, differentiation, and transplantation of stem cells to enhance their therapeutic advantages.

Despite the immense potential, problems in stem cell research for PD include assuring the survival, integration, and functionality of transplanted cells, as well as addressing potential ethical considerations connected with particular stem cell sources. However, improvements in induced pluripotent stem cells (iPSCs) and other ethical sources are minimizing these concerns, paving the way for more general acceptance and deployment of stem cell therapies in the treatment of PD.

As research in stem cell therapy continues, the objective is to produce a viable and scalable therapeutic option that can dramatically improve the lives of persons with PD, reducing or even arresting the progression of the illness.

Gene Therapy

Gene therapy is developing as a cutting-edge technique in the struggle against Parkinson's Disease, having the ability to treat the underlying genetic variables leading to the genesis and progression of the disorder. PD has a complicated genetic base, and gene therapy tries to repair or replace defective genes to restore normal cellular function.

In the context of PD, gene therapy frequently involves the delivery of therapeutic genes into specific parts of the brain, attempting to stimulate the production of critical proteins or regulate aberrant cellular processes. Viral vectors, such as adeno-associated viruses (AAVs), are routinely exploited to deliver therapeutic genes with precision. This tailored method minimizes off-target effects and enhances the specificity of treatment.

One of the interesting options in gene therapy for PD is the overexpression of proteins like GDNF (glial cell-derived neurotrophic factor), which has neuroprotective effects on dopamine-producing neurons. By boosting neuronal survival, gene therapy has the potential to delay or even reverse the degenerative process found in PD.

While gene therapy holds tremendous potential, obstacles include the requirement for accurate targeting, managing the degree of gene expression, and handling potential immunological responses. Ongoing research focuses on refining delivery systems, optimizing gene expression control, and ensuring long-term therapeutic effects.

In conclusion, the revolutionary approaches of Deep Brain Stimulation, Stem Cell Research, and Gene Therapy constitute formidable tools in the ongoing combat against Parkinson's Disease. As these medicines continue to grow and undergo rigorous research and clinical trials, they bring hope for more effective treatments and improved quality of life for persons living with PD.

CHAPTER SEVEN

PSYCHOSOCIAL SUPPORT FOR PATIENTS AND CAREGIVERS
Mental Health Considerations:

For patients and caregivers alike, the fight against Parkinson's disease is not just a physical one but also a significant emotional and mental one. For overall well-being, it is essential to identify and take care of the mental health issues related to Parkinson's disease. As they deal with the changes in their lives, patients frequently experience a range of emotions, such as worry, depression, and even bereavement.

Stress levels may rise as a result of the unknown nature of the disease's course and its effects on day-to-day functioning.

As they see their loved ones deal with the difficulties caused by Parkinson's, caregivers also experience a great deal of emotional strain. Because caring for someone else can be emotionally taxing, it's critical to recognize and meet their mental health requirements. Providing psychological support takes on a crucial role in the whole care plan, including counseling services and coping strategy tools. The inclusion of mental health specialists in the multidisciplinary team promotes resilience in the face of hardship and aids in the development of efficient coping strategies by patients and caregivers.

Education regarding the psychosocial elements of Parkinson's disease is also crucial. In addition to having the skills necessary to handle stress, anxiety, and depression, patients and caregivers must comprehend the possible effects of the illness on mental health. A more thorough and efficient strategy for treating Parkinson's disease involves creating a welcoming environment that promotes candid discussion about mental health issues.

Community Engagement and Support Groups:

It is impossible to overestimate the importance of a strong sense of community and shared experiences when overcoming Parkinson's disease's obstacles. For patients and caregivers alike, support groups are essential in giving them a feeling of community and understanding. By providing a forum for people to discuss their successes, failures, and insights, these groups help people build a supporting network outside of the hospital setting. Members of these groups receive helpful guidance on day-to-day living with Parkinson's disease in addition to emotional support.

Beyond support groups, community engagement encompasses a wider range of options. People with Parkinson's disease can better navigate the intricacies of the illness by having access to educational programs, workshops, and activities. Community involvement also aids in lowering isolation feelings, which are frequently connected to long-term medical conditions. Making relationships with people who are going through comparable things gives you a great support system and improves your quality of life.

In addition, Parkinson's disease awareness-raising community programs that involve patients and caregivers help to develop a feeling of purpose and advocacy. People who actively engage in activities and outreach initiatives become champions for their community and for themselves, which helps the overall effort to battle Parkinson's disease.

Keeping Help and Independence in Check:

A sensitive part of living with Parkinson's disease is knowing when to ask for help and when to keep yourself independent. As the illness worsens, people may find it harder to perform some tasks, so it's important to carefully assess whether and how to include help in day-to-day activities. Maintaining one's independence is essential for maintaining one's sense of self and identity, and medical professionals are essential in enabling patients to make knowledgeable decisions regarding their care.

When it comes to encouraging independence, adaptive techniques, and assistive technologies are useful instruments. These can include things like home changes that improve accessibility and safety or mobility assistance. Occupational therapy plays a crucial role in finding customized solutions that let patients carry out everyday duties more easily while maintaining their autonomy.

It is as crucial, though, to know when to accept help, though. To provide the required help without sacrificing the person's independence, caregivers frequently play a critical role. To ascertain the necessary degree of support and guarantee that it is in line with the patient's choices and objectives, open communication is crucial between patients, caregivers, and healthcare professionals.

Equally important is the psychological component of this balance. As the dynamics of independence and support change, patients may feel a variety of feelings, from annoyance to a sense of loss. It is imperative to confront these feelings and work together to find solutions that put the maintenance of an independent and satisfying life ahead of physical well-being. Parkinson's disease patients can manage this delicate balance while maximizing their overall quality of life by using a collaborative and person-centered approach.

CHAPTER EIGHT

COPING MECHANISMS FOR EVERYDAY LIFE
Adaptive Technology:

Adaptive technologies are unique as life-improving techniques in the field of managing Parkinson's disease. These devices are meant to fill the gap between the difficulties brought on by Parkinson's symptoms and the need for self-sufficiency. One such instance is wearable technology with motion sensors that monitor tremors and movements and provide caregivers and patients with immediate feedback. These advancements give people with Parkinson's disease the ability to keep an eye on their condition and give them a sense of control over their health.

Furthermore, sophisticated pharmaceutical administration systems have surfaced as a helpful tool for individuals managing intricate drug schedules linked to Parkinson's disease. These technologies ensure adherence and lower the chance of missed doses by providing reminders and dispensing medications at predetermined intervals. This relieves the strain on the individual and gives caregivers—who might be in charge of managing the pharmaceutical regimen—peace of mind.

Another essential adaptive technology that helps people with Parkinson's disease who have trouble speaking is speech recognition software. These apps help people communicate more effectively by turning spoken words into text, which makes it easier for people to express themselves.

This promotes independence while also assisting in the upkeep of social ties, which is essential for general well-being.

Essentially, as they provide useful answers to the day-to-day problems caused by the illness, adaptive technologies represent a dynamic frontier in the fight against Parkinson's. Despite the limitations of their condition, people can embrace a more independent and satisfying life by leveraging the power of invention.

Changes to a Home:

Adapting one's living environment becomes essential as Parkinson's disease advances to ensure safety, accessibility, and general well-being. Making changes to one's home is a proactive way to make the surroundings more suited to the special requirements of people with Parkinson's. Fall prevention is a major worry in Parkinson's care, and it can be greatly decreased with small changes like placing grab bars in convenient places and making sure the flooring is non-slip.

Additionally, by encouraging ease of mobility and reducing physical strain, ergonomic furniture, and fixtures can completely change living areas. For those with motor difficulties, everyday functioning is improved by taking into account elements like selecting furniture with supportive characteristics, modifying the height of counters, and laying out clear pathways. A sense of independence and confidence in one's ability to navigate one's own home is fostered by these improvements, which also solve immediate physical problems.

Another area of Parkinson's care that is experiencing change is home automation. Smart home technologies simplify activities like controlling lighting, thermostats, and even unlocking doors. They can be configured to react to voice requests or motion sensors. These changes make everyday routines easier to follow and less taxing physically on individuals.

All things considered, one of the main components of the integrative method of Parkinson's disease management is house changes. These modifications greatly improve quality of life and general well-being by modifying living spaces to meet people's changing needs.

Preserving Life Quality:

A person's and their support systems' primary concern when dealing with Parkinson's disease is preserving a high quality of life. Physical, emotional, and social well-being must all be considered in a multifaceted approach. Maintaining mobility and controlling symptoms are greatly aided by regular, capacity-appropriate physical activity. Exercise regimens that include cardiovascular, balancing, and flexibility exercises improve mental as well as physical wellness.

It is just as important to address emotional and psychological issues as physical wellness. Online or in-person support groups give people a place to talk about their experiences, coping mechanisms, and emotional support. In addition to helping people develop resilience and mental toughness, counseling services can be crucial in managing the emotional challenges brought on by a chronic illness.

A vibrant social life is essential to a high quality of life. Even if Parkinson's disease presents difficulties, loneliness can be mitigated by participating in hobbies, social activities, and community events. Like I said before, adaptive technologies help with this by making it easier to interact and communicate with friends and family.

In conclusion, a thorough and customized strategy is required to maintain a high quality of life while dealing with Parkinson's disease. People can traverse the intricacies of the disease with resilience and a sense of purpose by addressing the physical, emotional, and social elements. The fundamental importance of living a fulfilling life is emphasized by this holistic viewpoint, even when Parkinson's disease is present.

CHAPTER NINE

HOLISTIC METHODS FOR TREATING PARKINSON'S DISEASE
Complementary and Alternative Parkinson's Disease Therapies:

In addition to traditional medical treatments, complementary and alternative therapies are essential to the comprehensive care of patients with Parkinson's disease. These treatments seek to improve patients' quality of life, control symptoms, and promote general well-being. A famous method is acupuncture, an old Chinese treatment that involves putting tiny needles into particular body spots to ease pain and encourage balance. Research has indicated that acupuncture may be useful in treating

Parkinson's disease symptoms like rigidity and tremors.

Herbal medicine is another supplementary therapy gaining popularity. Because levodopa is a precursor to dopamine, some herbs, like Mucuna pruriens, have demonstrated promise in treating Parkinson's symptoms. Under the advice of medical specialists, some people include herbal supplements in their treatment regimen while research is still being done. Aromatherapy and massage treatment can also aid in relaxing and the alleviation of symptoms. While aromatherapy, which frequently uses essential oils, may have relaxing benefits on the nervous system, massage can assist in relieving tightness in the muscles and increase circulation.

It's important to remember that each person responds differently to complementary therapies, so it's important to talk to your healthcare physician to make sure these methods work with your patient's entire treatment plan. These treatments aim to provide a more thorough and individualized approach to

Parkinson's care, not to take the place of traditional medical measures.

Using Mind-Body Techniques to Manage Parkinson's Disease:

Integrative Parkinson's care emphasizes the connection between mental and physical health, and mind-body techniques are a key part of this. For example, mindfulness meditation has come to be recognized for its ability to improve one's sense of self and lower stress levels, both of which can be very helpful for those suffering from Parkinson's disease. Through encouraging present-moment awareness, mindfulness activities help people feel at ease and accepting of their circumstances.

Yoga is another mind-body technique that has demonstrated potential in the treatment of Parkinson's symptoms. Customized yoga practices can help with problems with strength, flexibility, and balance as well as with mobility and general physical function. Yoga offers a comprehensive approach to

Parkinson's care by fostering emotional well-being through the mind-body connection.

Furthermore, for Parkinson's sufferers, music therapy has become a cutting-edge mind-body intervention. Either actively playing an instrument or just listening to music, musical activities help improve motor abilities and emotional expression. Research findings suggest that listening to music with rhythmic auditory stimulation may aid in controlling movement patterns and lessen the severity of motor neurons.

Through the development of a sense of control and the promotion of general mental and physical health, these mind-body techniques enable people with Parkinson's disease to take an active role in their treatment. The therapy landscape for Parkinson's disease can be improved by incorporating these methods into an all-encompassing care plan.

Integrated Medicine in Comprehensive Parkinson's Disease Management:

From a holistic standpoint, integrative medicine treats Parkinson's disease by integrating alternative therapies and lifestyle changes with traditional medical treatments. This method acknowledges that treating a patient's emotional, social, and spiritual needs is just as important as treating their physical problems. By promoting cooperation between healthcare professionals, the integrative paradigm promotes a patient-centered approach to treatment.

One of the main focuses of integrative medicine for Parkinson's disease is nutritional therapy. A diet high in antioxidants and nutrients that is well-balanced can promote general health and possibly slow the course of a disease. Certain dietary regimens, including the Mediterranean diet, may have neuroprotective benefits and improve the prognosis of Parkinson's patients, according to some research.

Moreover, biofeedback and cognitive-behavioral therapy are two essential integrated care stress management strategies. Parkinson's symptoms can be made worse by long-term stress, therefore mastering these stress-reduction strategies can be beneficial to one's physical and emotional health. Integrative medicine also looks into the advantages of integrating exercise that is customized to each person's ability to increase mobility and functional independence.

Personalized care plans are critical in the field of integrative medicine. Healthcare professionals work in partnership with patients to customize interventions based on individual requirements, preferences, and goals, acknowledging that every person with Parkinson's disease is different. Recognizing the complexities of Parkinson's disease, this all-encompassing strategy aims to maximize the general health and quality of life of individuals afflicted with the illness.

CHAPTER TEN

INVESTIGATIONS AND UPCOMING PATHS
Clinical Trials And Ongoing Studies:

A wide range of active studies and clinical trials are characterizing the field of Parkinson's disease research, all of which are adding to the overall endeavor to comprehend, treat, and eventually eradicate this crippling neurological condition. To find new targets for intervention, several research projects are exploring the complex mechanisms underlying Parkinson's disease.

Thanks to developments in molecular biology, genetics, and neuroimaging, researchers can better understand the intricate interactions between environmental and genetic factors that lead to Parkinson's disease development and progression. These investigations hold great significance not only for expanding our comprehension of the illness but also for clearing the path for more potent therapies.

One of the most important stages in the process of translating knowledge into useful applications is clinical trials. Extensive testing is being done on experimental therapies, which include gene therapies and novel drugs, to assess their safety and effectiveness.

From individuals in the early stages of the disease to those with advanced stages, these studies include a wide range of participant demographics and offer important insights into how different treatments work at different points in the evolution of Parkinson's disease. A strong atmosphere for these trials is being created by cooperative efforts between academic institutions, pharmaceutical corporations, and patient advocacy groups.

This emphasizes the urgency and common commitment to discovering a treatment. The results of this research could transform the way that Parkinson's disease is treated, providing hope to millions of people who are impacted by the illness.

Potential Ground Breaks:

Recent years have seen encouraging discoveries in the field of Parkinson's disease research that are changing the course of potential treatments. For example, improvements in deep brain stimulation (DBS) methods have demonstrated impressive effectiveness in reducing motor symptoms and improving patients' quality of life.

Potential game-changers include the development of novel drug formulations and the repurposing of already-approved pharmaceuticals. To create more specialized and potent therapies, researchers are investigating cutting-edge strategies like focusing on particular proteins linked to Parkinson's pathology.

Furthermore, advances in precision medicine are enabling personalized therapeutic approaches based on patient characteristics, acknowledging the diversity of the Parkinson's community. Finding trustworthy markers of illness development and therapy response is the goal of the field of biomarker discovery, which is now receiving a lot of attention.

These discoveries help to the creation of disease-modifying treatments, which attempt to stop or slow down Parkinson's disease progression at its source in addition to providing hope for better symptom management.

Patient Input into Research:

It is impossible to overestimate the importance of patient advocacy in Parkinson's disease research since groups and individuals impacted by the illness actively shape the field's direction. To promote cooperation between scientists, physicians, and people with Parkinson's disease, patient advocacy groups are essential. The information is shared through these organizations, which guarantees that the needs and viewpoints of the Parkinson's community are taken into account when setting research priorities.

Instead of being passive recipients of research findings, patients, caregivers, and advocates actively participate in the planning, execution, and distribution of studies. Their personal experiences offer insightful information on the day-to-day difficulties brought on by Parkinson's disease and assist researchers in setting priorities for interventions that truly affect patients' quality of life.

Patient advocacy goes beyond setting research priorities; it also involves raising awareness, de-stigmatizing the condition, and arguing for laws that support funding for research and fair access to novel therapies. The Parkinson's community actively participates in research to ensure that it stays patient-centered and sensitive to the various needs of individuals affected by this neurological condition. As stakeholders, they have a vested interest in the outcomes of research activities.

CHAPTER ELEVEN

ACTIVATING THE PARKINSON'S DISEASE COMMUNITY
Awareness and Education:

One of the most important things that can be done to beat Parkinson's disease is to educate and raise awareness among those who live with the disease. With information about the illness, how it progresses, and the various available management techniques, education is a potent instrument for empowering people. It gives patients the knowledge they need to make wise decisions about their health and empowers them to take an active role in their treatment regimens.

Many topics should be covered in comprehensive training programs, such as the symptoms, the most recent research findings, and the scientific understanding of Parkinson's disease. This information helps patients, but it also helps caregivers and family members, building a community of understanding and support.

To ensure that this knowledge reaches a wider audience, workshops, webinars, and informational campaigns can be extremely important in spreading it.

Education should also go beyond the medical side of Parkinson's disease to include dietary advice, lifestyle changes, and mental health services. Education becomes a catalyst for better overall well-being by attending to the holistic requirements of people with Parkinson's disease. Programs that include patient testimonies and success stories have the potential to have a particularly large impact, providing hope and motivation to individuals facing the obstacles posed by the illness.

It is crucial to raise awareness on a larger scale in addition to schooling. This entails eradicating misconceptions and myths about Parkinson's disease, lowering stigma, and fostering understanding among the general public. The Parkinson's community can encourage empathy and gain public support by implementing focused awareness campaigns using a variety of media platforms. Parkinson's disease patients' overall well-being is greatly enhanced by the development of a more knowledgeable and caring society.

Promoting Changes in Policy:

Advocating for policy changes becomes crucial in the fight against Parkinson's disease since it calls for both systemic change and individual empowerment. To effect legislation, healthcare regulations, and research funds that directly affect the lives of those impacted by the disease, the Parkinson's community must actively interact with legislators and stakeholders.

Showcasing the special difficulties that people with Parkinson's disease and their families encounter is an essential part of effective advocacy. To improve knowledge and treatment choices, this involves promoting greater financing for Parkinson's research. It also means advocating for laws that guarantee everyone has access to high-quality medical care, including services specifically designed for people with Parkinson's disease.

To help people with Parkinson's disease keep their jobs and a sense of normalcy in their lives, it is also essential to advocate for workplace modifications and disability rights. Promoting laws that forbid discrimination and guarantee appropriate workplace modifications to meet the unique needs of people with Parkinson's disease is part of this.

Moreover, insurance coverage gaps and issues of affordability concerning Parkinson's care and treatment should be the focus of lobbying activities. Through proactive involvement with lawmakers, the Parkinson's community may strive for all-encompassing healthcare reform that takes into account the distinct requirements of people with chronic illnesses.

Advocating for policy changes is essentially a proactive, group endeavor to establish a supportive and elevating environment for the Parkinson's community. Ensuring that the perspectives of those impacted by Parkinson's are heard at all levels of decision-making, entails establishing bridges between patient advocacy organizations, medical experts, and legislators.

Creating a Helping Circle:

Creating an emotional, social, and practical support system for patients and their families is essential in the fight against Parkinson's disease. A strong support system includes peers, caregivers, community organizations, and medical professionals who specialize in Parkinson's disease.

Support groups are essential for connecting people with Parkinson's disease who are going through similar struggles. By offering a secure environment for exchanging advice, coping mechanisms, and experiences, these groups promote empathy and a sense of community.

Online platforms have the potential to augment the scope of support networks by enabling people to establish worldwide connections with one another, beyond geographical limitations.

Recognizing the critical role friends and family play in a person with Parkinson's disease journey, caregiver support is equally important. An atmosphere that fosters compassionate and sustainable caregiving is enhanced by caregiver tools and education, as well as the availability of respite care options.

Beyond personal relationships, Parkinson's support groups in the community can serve as focal points for advocacy, information, and resources. By fostering cooperation between patients, carers, and medical experts, these groups provide a broad network that meets the diverse requirements of the Parkinson's community.

Additionally, establishing alliances with local companies, employers, and educational institutions can help create a more welcoming atmosphere for people with Parkinson's disease. These collaborations help to create a supportive ecosystem that reaches beyond the local Parkinson's community by increasing awareness and fostering understanding in a variety of societal contexts.

In summary, assembling a cohesive web of linked assets and connections that uplift the Parkinson's community as a whole is the goal of developing a supportive network. It's a team effort that understands how crucial it is to have one another's back when facing the difficulties brought on by Parkinson's disease.